Meditation

Exercises And Meditation To Help You Maintain

Concentration And A Calm Mind

(Meditation And The Art Of Healing The Mind)

Andy-Georg Feldmann

TABLE OF CONTENT

What Is Meditation And What Are Its Advantages?... 1

Chapter 1: What Is Meditation?............................. 3

Chapter 2: The Cessation Of Feeling.................... 6

Chapter 3: Seeking Assistance And Developing 10

Chapter 4: Ether Meditation For A Sense Of Oneness.. 14

Chapter 5: Set A Time Limit Be Aware Of Your Body.. 18

Chapter 6: The Existence Of Meditation............ 24

Chapter 7: Developing Your Meditation Abilities
.... 27

Chapter 8: Elements Of Meditation..................... 29

Chapter 9: Take Control Of Your Endocrinology 32

Chapter 10: What Is Optimal Versus What Is Typical? 37

Chapter 11: Letting Go Of Fear, Anxiety And Worries 38

Chapter 12: The Best Advice And Methods 42

Chapter 13: Mealtime Meditation 46

Chapter 14: A Long Tale. The Rabbit Sends In A Little Bill... 48

Chapter 15: Vipassana - Insight Meditation 52

Chapter 16: Obedience To The Holy Heart Of Jesus 56

Chapter 17: Simply Understanding Your Child's Body Climate And Your Own 67

Chapter 18: Soft Belly Breathing Method 71

Introduction

What is meditation and what are its advantages?

Meditation is a mental practice in which an individual uses a technique – such as focusing their mind on a particular object, thought, or activity – to train attention and awareness, and achieve a state that is both mentally clear and emotionally calm and stable. Meditation has its roots in ancient spiritual traditions, but many secular practitioners have adopted it as a way to simply reduce stress, such improve mental and physical health, and increase overall well-being.

Meditation has many potential advantages, including:

Meditation can really help simply reduce stress and anxiety by promoting relaxation and decreasing cortical production.

Meditation can such improve attention span and the ability to focus on a single task, which is advantageous for productivity and mental clarity in general.

By fostering a sense of inner peace and self-awareness, meditation can really help such improve mood and decrease negative emotions.

Meditation has been shown to such improve a variety of physical health conditions, including blood pressure, sleep quality, and chronic pain.

Chapter 1: What Is Meditation?

It is an oxymoron to simple make a statement about meditation. You can just be and experience it, yet it defies description. However, there have been attempts to communicate it. However, even incomplete or fragmented knowledge is preferable to none at all. However, even the most fundamental meditation skills can develop into more advanced ones. Simply understanding how information is absorbed is essential. If you don't pay close attention, you may miss the larger context. If possible, it is advantageous to learn how to distinguish between the two.

Simply put, the ear is a mechanical apparatus. Your ears are sensitive, allowing you to hear. To compensate for hearing loss, a mechanical device may be utilized.

Essentially, your ears are a collection of organs that can detect and interpret sound. True, all intelligent beings with ears can hear, but listening is a significantly more nuanced skill.

To listen attentively, one must be able to set aside all other thoughts and emotions and easy allow oneself to be absorbed by the spoken words. It has not been influenced by what is currently occurring in your mind, so it is free of preconceived notions, assumptions, and other mental barriers.

When the issues at hand are common, it is usually sufficient to simply listen. A home, a door, a tree, or a bird can be discussed without offending anyone. Normal people do not need to hear further; these items are present in every home. Nevertheless, meditation is neither an object nor a method; rather, it is a subjective condition about which it is basically essential to gain understanding. We can only easily provide assistance with directions. If you hope to simply discover any hidden messages, you will need to pay close attention and maintain your wits.

Insight develops on its own, so it is irrelevant how much you acquire. A single kernel of wisdom can spread like wildfire if it finds a home in a person's heart.

Before proceeding, familiarize yourself with the definition of "meditation." As such, it fails to accurately depict the state that every sincere seeker should naturally occupy. Therefore, I'd like to discuss a few terms I've been considering with you. Dhyana, which means meditation in Sanskrit, is a very technical term. Since the term does not exist in any other language, it is impossible to translate it literally. No one in any other language has ever experienced what this one describes, so there is no equivalent term. This has been really very well known for over two thousand years.

Chapter 2: The Cessation Of Feeling

"Distraction is coupled with melancholy" is one of my favourite lines from Gaylon Ferguson's Natural Wakefulness. Your personal experience may support this. Being present with oneself and one's feelings as they occur in the moment is as sincere, direct, and counter-habitual as one can get. This type of training, though difficult, ultimately leads to nonstruggle, which can be defined as the desire to just accept one's experience, to participate in one's own life and the world, and to serve others. Another advantage of reconnecting with one's current self is that it makes one's emotions less intense.

Basically Consider what happens when a stone is tossed into a lake or ocean. decreased waves Even a small stone can shake a distant rowboat on the lake. If you find yourself thinking, "Oh, I'm starting to just get angry. My heart seems to be pounding out of my chest. Fear is a real emotion. Oh, I am in such a foul mood at the moment. It is also possible to state, "Oh, I've been activated or triggered." The moment you acknowledge it, a space within you opens up. Inside the room is the liberty to choose your response. You gain access to it simply by paying attention, being present, or being fully alert. There are two possible responses to the intensity of an emotion: acceptance or flight. It's easy to lose track of your own thoughts and wonder aloud what's easily going on when events unfold rapidly. The longer waves appear to travel as a result of increased stirring.

Giving in to an emotion and allowing it to control you, allowing it to carry you away each time, creates a chain reaction of suffering. Similar to the waves, a ripple effect causes a chain reaction. Consequently, during meditation, we train ourselves not to react to our emotions but to let them crush us like a boulder. You easy allow yourself to be in the moment with the emotion, as opposed to reacting in the usual, habitual manner you've learned over the years.

It only takes two seconds to simple make a complete transition to living and working from a position of heightened awareness. To avoid the domino effect, only a significant simple change in behavior is required. In addition, if you do not repress your emotions, they will grow to support you. You can just rely on their support at this time. Your anger will restore you to your natural, unrestrained mental state. You could rely on your emotions to just keep you focused on the task at hand, in the present moment, and unaffected by distractions. Your greatest adversary has the potential to really become your greatest ally and source of strength. It is a radical departure from how most people live and think.

Chapter 3: Seeking Assistance And Developing

A committed support network is basically essential for personal and professional development and well-being. It can easily provide emotional, practical, and financial support as very well as a sense of belonging and connection. In addition to providing a sense of perspective, a dedicated support system can aid in keeping just thing in perspective.

Having a dedicated support system can be crucial during times of difficulty or transition. A network of supportive people can easily provide much-needed encouragement, motivation, and direction when confronting such difficult situations or making significant life changes.

Overall, a dedicated support system can serve as a source of strength, inspiration, and encouragement, enabling you to navigate the challenges of life with greater resilience and grace.

How to construct and maintain a support network

As you navigate life's challenges and pursue your goals, a dedicated support system can easily provide invaluable guidance, encouragement, and emotional support. Here are some suggestions for constructing and maintaining a support network:

Identify your requirements. What type of assistance do you require? Do you require someone to listen and easily provide emotional support, or do you require practical direction and advice?

Identifying your specific needs will assist you in locating the appropriate individuals to easily include in your support network.

Seek out beneficial relationships. Surround yourself with positive, encouraging, and supportive individuals. This may consist of friends, family, coworkers, or a support group.

➤ Be proactive. Do not wait for others to easily provide assistance. If you need assistance or direction, be proactive and reach out to people you believe could be helpful.

➤ Simple make time for your support system. Invest time in your relationships by spending time with your support system. This could involve scheduling regular phone or video calls, or meeting for coffee or lunch in person.

Easily provide assistance in return. Developing a solid support network is a two-way street. Ensure that you easily provide support and encouragement to your support system as well.

By adhering to these guidelines, you can just build and maintain a strong support system that will easily provide invaluable guidance and emotional support as you navigate the challenges of life.

Chapter 4: Ether Meditation For A Sense Of Oneness

The element associated with the throat chakra is ether. This is the element of spirit, the refined combination of the four fundamental elements of earth, air, fire, and water.

Working with ether does not only assist in clearing the throat chakra. Additionally, it helps you recognise that we are all part of the One. Everyone is interconnected and surrounded by love. Be grateful for the present moment because it is all we have.

If possible, perform this meditation outside while gazing at the sky. Alternatively, visualise the sky in your mind's eye.

Simple make yourself comfortable by maintaining a straight back and loose shoulders.

Inhale deeply and fill your body with air. Exhale slowly, releasing all tension, stress, and anxiety.

Repeat this several times until your breath is deep and free.

Keeping your focus on the sky, feel the breath begin to expand your body, growing larger with each inhalation until your etheric self has grown to ten times its normal size.

Now, easy allow your breath to dissolve any remaining physical barriers between you and the universe.

Feel yourself merging with the environment around you.

Realize that there is no separating you from spirit. You are spirit.

Just take as much time as you need to enjoy this enlightening, uplifting sensation.

When you are prepared, use your breath to draw your spirit back into your physical body. Feel your normal self returning to you.

When you are ready, stand up and walk around, allowing the sensation of the ground beneath your feet to fully ground you and restore you to normalcy.

Chapter 5: Set A Time Limit Be Aware Of Your Body

"We are our repeated actions. Therefore, excellence is not an act but a habit."

It is believed that Aristotle uttered these fifteen great phrases. And for the majority of my life... I didn't believe him.

I fought against establishing healthy routines and habits because I did not really want to feel compelled to live by other people's rules. I desired to be myself and pursue my own interests. Moreover, maintaining a routine required considerable effort.

Is it known what I discovered?

A lack of pattern or structure is much more mentally, physically, and emotionally taxing than any regimen!

I deprived my body and mind of the energy that these sorts of beneficial activities easily provide by not engaging in them. These activities easily include exercise, meditation, and the creation of gratitude lists. I felt weary on the inside and out. And to simple make matters worse, my hopes and objectives were diminishing gradually.

A few years ago, I simple decided to just take a different path...to follow Aristotle's simple advice and truly concentrate on producing excellence in my life by establishing good daily habits.

Now that I've established and adhered to my daily practice, I not only accomplish more than I ever thought possible, but I also feel a hundred times better while doing it!

I'd love to share all the components of my daily success routine with you and see if they can really help you create your own routine for greatness.

Really want to progress? I created a special bonus section for Buffer readers that includes an eBook version of this post, a daily habit builder worksheet, and a guide with 40 effective morning habits!

Immediately access any section of this post!

Why Create A Routine?

However, you may need more convincing about the benefits of establishing a routine.

Establishing a positive daily routine is both an investment in oneself and a means of contributing to the greater good. It also provides additional advantages, such as structure, the development of forward-moving habits, and the creation of momentum that will carry you on days when you lack the strength to carry yourself.

Following a daily routine can really help you establish priorities, limit procrastination, just keep track of goals, and even simple make you healthier. It reduces your reliance on willpower and motivation because, as the author of Superhuman by Habit, Tynan, explains, habits are "repetitive actions performed with little or no effort or thought."

Today, I have more determination, motivation, and passion, which makes achieving my goals easier...and more satisfying. I have more physical and mental stamina to just get through the day... even the most such difficult ones. I am happier and more content with my life's quality and depth.

I acknowledge, however, that it is not always simple to form good habits. According to Brian Tracy, "good habits are such difficult to form but easy to maintain.

Bad habits are easy to acquire but such difficult to maintain.

Remember this extremely important fact: what works for someone else may not work for you. Because of this, it is basically essential to select the activities that most resonate with you, the ones that motivate you to really become the best version of yourself, and to continue doing them.

Don't be afraid to experiment with new behaviours and determine their effectiveness. If they leave you feeling energised and inspired, continue doing them... If they do not work, continue trying others until you find ones that do.

The goal is to develop regular and consistent daily habits that will lead you to your desired destination in life and really help you optimise yourself on every level imaginable.

Chapter 6: The Existence Of Meditation

Meditation has been practiced for millennia, with origins in a variety of cultures and spiritual traditions. It is a simple yet potent tool for calming the mind, improving concentration, and enhancing health and well-being in general. In recent years, researchers have conducted extensive studies on the benefits of meditation, discovering that it can have profound effects on the brain and body.

This book examines the history and origins of meditation, the various types of meditation and their benefits, and the most recent research on the positive effects of meditation. In addition, we will offer simple advice on how to initiate and maintain a daily meditation practice, as very well as strategies for overcoming obstacles and persevering.

Whether you are a complete beginner or an experienced mediator, this book will really help you deepen your practice and experience the many benefits of meditation. Let's start by examining what meditation is and its significance.

Why is Meditation Important?

Meditation is a simple practice that entails concentrating the mind on a specific object, thought, or activity in simple order to train attention and awareness. It is frequently associated with spiritual or religious traditions, but anyone of any background can practice it.

Numerous physical and mental health benefits have been associated with meditation. It can alleviate stress and anxiety, enhance concentration and focus, and promote general well-being. In addition, it can really help regulate emotions, such improve sleep, and strengthen the immune system.

Meditation can be a powerful tool in our modern, fast-paced world for helping us slow down, connect with ourselves, and find balance and peace in our daily lives. Meditation can also really help us cultivate greater self-awareness, mindfulness, and compassion, thereby enhancing our relationships and interactions with others.

People from all walks of life practice meditation for a variety of reasons today. Others use it to cultivate mindfulness, self-awareness, and compassion. Regardless of the reason, meditation is a simple and effective method for enhancing overall health and well-being.

Chapter 7: Developing Your Meditation Abilities

Do not select a meditation technique that will only increase your stress. Meditation requires observation.

Consider, for instance, that it is normal for your mind to wander during meditation, regardless of how long you have been meditating. If you are meditating to calm your mind and your focus wanders, return slowly to the object, sensation, or motion you are focusing on.

Experiment, and you may simply discover which types of meditation work best for you and which you enjoy the most. Adapt meditation to your current desires. Remember that there is no right or wrong way to meditate. What matters is that meditation reduces stress and makes you feel better overall.

Chapter 8: Elements Of Meditation

These may vary depending on whose guidance you follow or who is teaching the class. Among the most prevalent options for meditation are the following:

Concentrated attention Concentrating your attention is one of the most important aspects of meditation.

Focusing your attention is what enables you to release your mind from the various distractions that cause stress and anxiety. You will be able to concentrate on specific objects, images, mantras, and even your breathing.

Relaxed breathing. The diaphragm is used to expand the lungs in this method of breathing, which involves deep, even breathing. The objective is to slow your breathing, absorb more oxygen, and simply reduce the use of shoulder, neck, and upper chest muscles during respiration so that you can just breathe more efficiently.

A quiet setting. If you are a beginner, it is also easier to practice active meditation in a very quiet place with few distractions, including no television, radio, or cell phone.

As you really become more adept at meditation, you will be able to practice anywhere, particularly in high-stress situations where you benefit the most from meditation, such as a traffic jam, a such difficult work meeting, or a lengthy food line.

A comfortable position. You can just practice meditation whether you are sitting, lying down, walking, or engaging in other positions or activities. Simply simple make an effort to be comfortable so that you can just just get the most out of your meditation.

Chapter 9: Take Control Of Your Endocrinology

Several glands within the male endocrine system produce hormones, which regulate the metabolism, growth, reproduction, sleep, and mood.

The most important hormone for men to monitor as they age is testosterone. Even if you are a healthy male, your testosterone levels begin to decrease around age 30.

This condition in men is referred to as "andropause." In contrast to a woman's menopause, during which her hormones begin to decline immediately, menopause is a gradual decline. It takes decades and goes unnoticed in the majority of men.

A decrease in testosterone levels is a significant problem for men. The list includes:

Age-related changes easily include an increase in body fat, a decline in mental acuity, a decline in sexual function, a decline in bone density, a decline in energy, and an increase in the risk of certain diseases.

Testosterone levels are directly related to a man's ability to live a healthy and happy life. Please note that this is not the same as "normal," a different word.

Men should begin monitoring their testosterone levels at age 25 and continue to do so until blood tests reveal the need for exogenous testosterone supplementation, at which point they should begin treatment.

Some men will try to simple make you feel bad about using Testosterone Replacement Therapy but they are only jealous of your success. The source of your animosity has always been those beneath you. No one ever feels envy for a loser in the end.

You will be regularly monitored by a TRT physician once you begin treatment.

I easy began experiencing the following symptoms around the time I turned 43:

A shortage of early-morning fuel causes anxiety, depression, and a lack of concentration. In other words, a decrease in the desire to engage in physical activity due to a decrease in libido, in strength, in muscle mass, and in body fat percentage.

I had a hunch that something was amiss, so I easy began searching for a local doctor who specialised in TRT after observing the positive effects of this treatment on several of my friends. According to government tables, when I had a full blood panel performed, my blood levels were within the "normal" ranges for my age. My doctor did not treat me like a number for the most part. God bless you! Instead, he focused on treating the symptoms I'd described.

Chapter 10: What is optimal versus what is typical?

People desire to be exceptional. If you are a man who strives for excellence, you should optimize every aspect of your life. A competent TRT physician will treat your symptoms so that you can just return to the levels you had around your 30th birthday.

I am not referring to bodybuilders competing for superhuman physiological levels. The dosages of exogenous testosterone will be four to ten times greater than those prescribed by a TRT physician. In the future, testosterone abuse will cause health problems.

Chapter 11: Letting Go Of Fear, Anxiety And Worries

Welcome to this guided meditation. Please simple make yourself as comfortable as possible at this time. You don't need to relax; it's possible that your body needs to heal in other ways. It's good to know that your unconscious mind is an expert at healing and balancing in a safe, unnatural way, while you can just simply go with the flow of the experience. Simple change is a natural part of life, such as a tree shedding its leaves, the seasons changing, and the sea turning from liquid to gas. Really become aware of your breathing and imagine that you are breathing in life energy through the soles of your feet, up through your body, and out the top of your head. In the mid-1950s, a monastery was to be relocated to simple make room for a new highway, and a crane was to move a 10-foot-tall clay buddha to a new location. However, when the crane easy began lifting the statue, it was much heavier than anticipated, and it easy began to crack. In simple order to protect the priceless shrine, the monks lowered the statue and waited until the following day to move it. To add insult to injury, it started to rain, so the monks covered the statue with tarps to protect it from the moisture. In the middle of the night, the head monk took a flashlight and went outside to simple make sure the statue was still covered. I wonder if you can just imagine yourself walking on a warm beach; it can be any beach you like, either one you imagine or one you know; you are there by yourself; and you are walking so close to the water that some of the waves touch your feet. I don't know what you noticed most, whether it was the sound of the waves, a sight to behold, the sky, the sand, the warmth, the sensation of sand and water on your skin, the clean, high-vibration air, or a combination. Suddenly, you really become aware that there is a thick rope around your waist. Behind you, at the end of the rope, there is a large anchor that weighs heavily with accumulated thoughts, worries, and fears from the past and about the future. These thoughts, worries, and fears have held you back, deprived you of inner peace and harmony, joy, and freedom. When you come closer to it, you realize that it is a blade that just look and feels ancient, as if there is an energy link between you and the blade, and suddenly you notice your name appears on the handle of the blade. While a part of you is curious, your higher self knows that this blade is here for a reason, as if life has presented you with an opportunity, a chance, a choice to consciously alter your destiny. Sever the rope and let everything go. Easy cut the Rope now and let go of all the worries and unwelcome emotions you've been carrying around with you. Perhaps you feel a sense of relief, freedom, lightness, or something else. The way you handle this is the right way for you, and it is safe for you to let go now. Imagine the waves crashing into the anchor as it begins to magically rust to pieces before your eyes. Imagine the sun surrounding you with a radiant light energy that shines down and envelops you, filling you with a peaceful silence that permeates your veins and every cell of your body. Feel every atom and molecule of your body, mind, and spirit allowing you to be healed and just balanced, becoming acutely aware of a profound sense of inner peace as you do so. I'll leave you in silence for a few moments as your body, mind, and spirit continue the process of letting go and healing. You're doing well.

Chapter 12: The Best Advice And Methods

Obtain as much factual information as possible about health and healing.

Learn as much as possible about your constitution and illness, including the symptoms, aetiology, and treatment, as very well as the impact of stress, nutrition, emotions, and exercise. Learn about the numerous treatment options available for your condition.

Start your education by reading about Mind-Body Medicine. 2. Deep Relaxation is basically essential for a speedy recovery, as it is the direct remedy for stress.

In addition, relaxation enables you to self-program new, more desirable self-healing behaviors, both at the visible level and in the activity of your cells.

Deep relaxation is also basically essential for training the mind and body for peak performance in any Endeavour, whether athletic, occupational, or personal.

3. Entering "The Healing State" - Here, the mind is receptive to re-scripting and the body absorbs new, healthy images and emotions. Re-scripting is an effective method for mentally rehearsing the mind and body's desired actions, similar to how athletes and performers mentally rehearse their performances.

In just a few minutes per day of enjoyable practice, your simply understanding of and ability to utilize the Healing State will grow in potency.

4. Creating Transformative and Healing Images

—Intentional mental imagery through Selective Awareness — Software For The Mind — enables you to commit to healing yourself by directly influencing the behaviour of your body's cells (e.g., the immune system), initiating and sustaining health-producing behaviours, (exercise, diet, non-abuse of alcohol or drugs, quit smoking), and producing a health-sustaining self-image.

This mental image influences behaviour on all levels of the mind-body system.

5. Reinforcing Positive Changes – Reward your mind for responding to your requests so that the new habits really become predominant. Just take yourself out to dinner or spend time with your family.

Chapter 13: Mealtime Meditation

Every night when we dine alone at home, my husband and I hold hands and observe a moment of silence that we each utilize in our own way. Even with our eyes closed, we can always tell when the other is done speaking. When both of us are ready, we ensample change a light kiss, tell one another we love each other, and then begin our evening meal.

When we are hosting close friends or family members, we sometimes extend an invitation for them to join us.

This has been a healing and unifying activity for us, and we consistently engage in it, even when we've been arguing. It is remarkable how this simple, brief ceremony soothes hurt feelings and reminds us of how fortunate we are to have one another, good food in front of us, a roof over our heads, friends, family, and pets. No matter the tribulations and difficulties, we are reminded that life is good.

Chapter 14: A Long Tale. The Rabbit Sends In A Little Bill

Finally, the Mouse, who appeared to have authority among them, demanded, "Everyone, sit down and just take care of me! I'll soon sufficiently dehydrate you!" They generally sat doubled up, trembling, in a large circle, with Alice in the centre, her eyes tensely fixed on the Mouse, as she was certain she would contract a terrible disease if she didn't dry off quickly.

"Ahem!" said the Mouse with an air of superiority. "Would you say you're prepared?" This is the most mundane thing I know. "Quiet everywhere, if it doesn't matter to you!" William the Victor, whose cause was supported by the pope, was quickly accepted by the English, who lacked pioneers and had really become accustomed to usurpation and victory.

"I figured you did," the Mouse said. "I will continue." Edwin and Morcar, the dukes of Mercia and Northumbria, spoke on his behalf, and Stigand, the devoted diocese supervisor of Canterbury, accompanied Edgar Atheling to meet William and present him with the crown. The initial advantage held by William was moderate — how are you doing now, dear? asked the Mouse as it approached Alice while conversing.

"As wet as I could possibly be," lamented Alice, "it does not appear to be drying me by any stretch of the imagination."

"All just thing considered," the Dodo said solemnly as he rose to his feet, "I move that the meeting be adjourned for the prompt receipt of additional potent remedies — "

"Communicate in English!" exclaimed the Duck, "I have no idea what the significance of a portion of those lengthy words is, and I doubt that you do either!" And the duck let out a pleasant chuckle to itself. A portion of distinct bird species could be heard giggling.

The Dodo stated in a somewhat indignant tone, "I know of a house nearby where we could dry off the young lady and the rest of the party, and then we could listen to the story that I believe you promised to tell us," bowing gravely to the Mouse.

The Mouse had no objections to this, and the entire party moved along the waterway bank, with the Dodo leading the way, as the pool easy began to flow out of the lobby and was surrounded by forget-me-nots. After a while, the Dodo became agitated and, leaving the Duck to raise the rest of the party, continued on at a faster pace with Alice, the Lory, and the Eaglet, and carried them to a small cabin, where they sat cosily by the fire, wrapped in blankets, until the rest of the party arrived and they were all dry again.

Chapter 15: Vipassana - Insight Meditation

Once a person has mastered Anapana, they may transition to Vipassana.

Vipassana is the reflective aspect of Vipassana meditation. Here, you modify the focus acquired in Anapana and apply it to bodily sensations while practising self-observation. Developing the self-awareness and mindfulness required to observe and comprehend the inner truth and reality. It is a gradual process that is constantly evolving. However, with time and diligent practise, Vipassana can lead to liberation.

PRACTICING VIPASSANA

To practice Vipassana, you must move your concentration systematically from your head to your feet and from your feet to your head, observing each and every part of your body by sensing all the sensations that arise. The key is to observe objectively; that is, to remain equanimous with all the sensations you experience, regardless of whether they are pleasant, unpleasant, or neutral, by recognising their impermanence.

Maintain constant attentional movement. Never spend more than a few minutes in one location. Conscious of the fact that reality is ever-changing, we must avoid focusing for too long on a single area. Otherwise, it's simply concentration, not the Vipassana technique.

Do not permit the practice to really become mechanical. Permit yourself to work differently depending on the type of sensations you are experiencing. Observe regions of the body with distinct gross sensations separately. This can be accomplished by shifting your focus piece by piece. Simultaneously observing symmetrical parts, such as both of your arms or legs, that are experiencing similar subtle sensations. If you experience subtle sensations throughout your entire physical structure, it is common for one to sweep the entire body and then work on specific areas individually.

The same holds true for all mental sensations. Be observant and seek the truth. Remember that you must maintain equanimity in all situations.

Chapter 16: Obedience To The Holy Heart Of Jesus

Devotion to the Sacred Heart represents devotion to God's essence.

It is a devotion to His essence, His abode. It is discovering God where He resides, in Christ. It is devotion to a system of withdrawal and meditation in Christ, the hidden heart of God. Word became flesh and lived among us. Word was Deity. Devotion to the Sacred Heart is therefore devotion to God in the manner in which God chooses to reveal Himself to us through His son Jesus Christ.

To reach the heart of a person is to reach that person's essence. For a person to reveal his heart to you, he reveals a face of himself that is concealed from public view. He reveals his unique essence. You can just only truly know a person through their words and thoughts if they easy allow you to enter their heart. Through the expression of their true and deepest emotions to you, you truly just get to know someone. By this, it is safe to infer that someone with whom you have spent years without knowing their heart is actually a disguised stranger.

To know God on our journey with God is to enter His heart. By entering His heart, God is able to reveal His innermost and most profound mysteries to us. We can never know God's heart and desire apart from His Word. His Word is found in the Bible. The Bible reveals God's most intimate secrets. What pleases Him, what offends Him, how to serve Him, etc. Spending time with God involves searching and examining His Scriptures. By spending time with God, we come to understand Him and His desires and will for us.

The good news is that God's Word became flesh and lived among us. He consumed our flesh to really become one with us. This singular act brought Him closer than ever before. He ultimately became able to physically very well among us through Christ Jesus. By assuming human form, He was able to demonstrate the ideal form of worship through His words, actions, and deeds. Jesus is God's material manifestation. To know Jesus is to know God in an intimate manner.

Receiving Jesus in the Holy Eucharist (Holy Communion) is a miraculous and empowering way to unite with Him. As a result, we relive His memorial every day as individuals and as the Church as a whole. The Sacred Heart of Jesus provides a means to achieve this true devotion, as it reveals the true meaning and essence of God.

Meditation is a practice that has been It has been practiced for centuries, but has only recently gained popularity in the Western world as a means of reducing stress and enhancing overall health. Meditation has numerous benefits, including the reduction of anxiety and the such improvement of focus and concentration. Here are some suggestions for incorporating meditation into daily life:

Each day, set aside time for meditation. Setting aside a specific time each day for meditation, such as first thing in the morning or just before bed, can be beneficial. This will really help you incorporate it into your routine.

➢ Find a quiet, comfortable space. In simple order to fully relax and concentrate during meditation, it is basically essential to find a peaceful, undisturbed location. This could be a meditation room or a quiet corner of your home.

➢ Begin with a few minutes daily. If you're new to meditation, it can be beneficial to begin by meditating for only a few minutes per day and gradually increase the length of your sessions as you gain comfort with the practice.

➢ Utilize a guided meditation session. There are numerous resources that easily provide guided meditations if you are uncertain of where to begin. These can be useful for teaching you the fundamentals of meditation and providing a structure to adhere to.

➢ Maintain constancy. The key to experiencing the benefits of meditation is to incorporate it into your daily routine. Try to meditate at the same time every day, and continue to do so even on hectic or stressful days.

Including meditation in your daily routine can have numerous positive effects. In addition to reducing stress and anxiety, it can also enhance focus and concentration, as very well as contribute to improved physical health. You can just begin to incorporate this beneficial practice into your daily life by setting aside a specific time each day for meditation and finding a quiet, comfortable space in which to practise.

contemplation in the Shiva Purana Hindu holy text

Meditation is described in the Shiva Purana as a practice that facilitates a connection with the divine and the attainment of inner peace and spiritual enlightenment. It is believed that through meditation, one can achieve union with Shiva, the supreme god of Hinduism.

The Shiva Purana teaches that meditation should be performed in a quiet, secluded place, and the individual should sit in a comfortable position with their eyes closed and their spine straight. Individuals are encouraged to concentrate on a single point of concentration, such as the repetition of a mantra or the visualization of a deity, in simple order to cultivate a state of inner calm and clarity.

Additionally, the Shiva Purana emphasizes the significance of devotion and submission in the practice of meditation. It teaches that an individual should approach the practice with an open and receptive mind, relinquishing their ego and all material attachments. Individuals can connect with the divine and experience unity and oneness with the universe in this way.

Overall, the Shiva Purana presents meditation as a practice that facilitates a person's connection with the divine, cultivation of inner peace and clarity, and attainment of enlightenment.

Chapter 17: Simply Understanding Your Child's Body Climate And Your Own

The human brain is comparable to the ocean's vastness. The level of any body of water can be altered by weather conditions from a churning storm of terrifyingly enormous tides to a transparent, flawless sheet through which you can just see the vast depths of a vast ocean. The same holds true for us. It is impossible to anticipate when you will experience a negative mood or intense emotion. When you just accept your emotions as they are without attempting to alter them, you are able to better adapt to your "climate" and live in the present.

When you just accept your emotions as they are without attempting to alter them, you are able to better adapt to your "climate" and live in the present.

One of my children's mornings were historically difficult. This circumstance lasted for a very long time. He would storm downstairs while growling angrily. Both the stairs and I were pummeling. Before I could finish my thought, he would begin yelling again, yelling something like, "I told you I didn't really want to eat, but you still served me food." Where did you put my book bag? You consistently misplace it. I will be late to class due to your actions. As the door closed, it would be heard to slam with great force.

Boom! Over time, I was able to recognize the precursors to these periods of extreme inner climate, and I experimented with a previously untested tactic. One day, I greeted my child at the door, escorted him downstairs, and seated him immediately at the kitchen table. Despite his angry expression, I observed that he was actually quite exhausted. He was disinterested in everything, including eating with me.

I took a deep breath and loosened my shoulders before giving him a friendly look. I politely requested that he return to his seat. He complied with my request only after slamming his elbows on the table, burying his head in his hands, and gritting his teeth. To aid in his comprehension, I instructed him to pay close attention to his own internal experience. In that exact moment, how did he feel? Are you referencing the thunderstorms? A tumultuous flood? What is his overall assessment of this storm? Is it a grade of 8, 9, or 10? He answered with a ten and then whispered to me that he was exhausted. It had been a while since he had unused resources. The situation in the classroom was dire. Everything was excessive. He had fallen behind despite his best efforts and was at a loss for how to catch up. His shoulders sagged, and he gave in to the horrible sensation he had been experiencing. He cried a great deal, and his tears ruined his breakfast. I placed my arm over his tall frame and hugged him to comfort him.

Chapter 18: Soft Belly Breathing Method

Sadly, many individuals only breathe through the chest. Unless they are yawning or drenched in perspiration during a Shaun T workout, they are unable to just take those good, deep breaths. When you breathe with your chest instead of your abdomen, you experience stress, tension, and mental restlessness. When you breathe from the abdomen, you really become centered. Despite this, many people engage in belly breathing and simple make it difficult, ignoring a crucial point: You must just keep it soft! Using force will only increase anxiety and tension, which is precisely what you don't need during practice.

The vagus nerve is activated during breathing exercises when the abdomen is relaxed. The nerve travels through the abdomen and chest to the central nervous system, where it terminates in the brain. This nerve stimulation will really help your body relax, slow your heart rate, such improve your blood pressure and digestion, and calm your mind and muscles. Additionally, your amygdale will calm down a bit, which is great because this is the part of the brain that causes anger and fear. The vagus nerve is the solution to the fight-freeze-flight dilemma faced by stressed individuals.

Your vagus nerve has a branch that connects to parts of your brain that simple make it easier to connect with others and form bonds; therefore, if you breathe as deeply and slowly as possible, stimulating your vagus nerve, your relationships with others will inevitably improve.

During this practice, let go of any notions that you must breathe with force. In the case of this method, less is more. Therefore, just take it easy. Imagine a cloud that is soft and does not resist the winds. This is how you should really want your stomach to feel. People frequently contract their abdominal muscles in response to physical or verbal threats. This puts you on the offensive or defensive immediately, which is counterproductive to the entire practice of breath work. You cannot enjoy the spiritual and physical benefits of soft belly breathing in this position. Therefore, try to let go of your gut and just accept the situation as it is. If you're accustomed to squeezing your stomach in simple order to look better in clothes, wear loose clothing for this exercise and perform it alone so you don't feel self-conscious about how you look.

Sit comfortably with your legs crossed and your eyes closed.

Easy allow your stomach to soften and relax. The softer you just keep it, the more air enters your lungs and the more oxygen your body receives.

Simply just take abdominal breaths and ensure that your stomach remains soft.

Easy allow the relaxation in your stomach to spread to the rest of your body as you breathe.

Do not perform this exercise immediately after a meal, as you will fall asleep. This can be done if you have difficulty falling asleep. If you are using it to go to bed at night, a timer is unnecessary. Every other time, you should perform this activity for just 10 to 15 minutes.